Stay
Healt
Alfred E
2023

Did You Eat Your Vitamins Today?

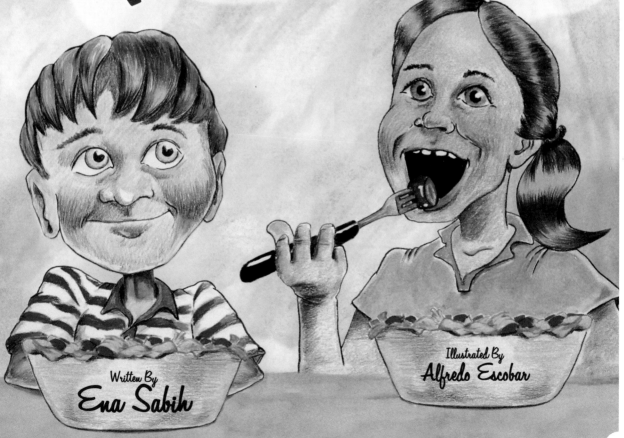

Written By
Ena Sabih

Illustrated By
Alfredo Escobar

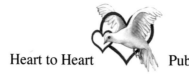

Heart to Heart Publishing, Inc.

Heart to Heart Publishing, Inc.
528 Mud Creek Road • Morgantown, KY 42261
(270) 526-5589
www.hearttoheartpublishinginc.com

Printed in Canada
Friesens
Manitoba, Canada

Copyright 2010 Ena Sabih
Publishing Date: January 2011
Library of Congress: 2010942850
ISBN 978-0-9802486-7-8

Editor: Lou Beeker Schultz
Co-Editor: L. J. Gill
Proofreader: Evelyn Byers
Illustrator: Alfredo Escobar
Designer: April S. Yingling

This book was written to educate children about the role of vitamins and to generate an interest in healthy foods. The information and vocabulary used in this book have been greatly simplified for the understanding of young children, and it does not include complete information on the uses and effects of vitamins. Some of the foods mentioned in this book may not be suitable for all children (or adults), given their specific age and health conditions.

The information in this book is for educational purposes only and is not intended to suggest, recommend, or replace any medical advice. All matters concerning health should be addressed and supervised by a licensed and qualified health professional. The author and publisher assume no responsibility for any adverse effects or consequences arising, directly or indirectly, from the use or application of any information contained in this book.

FSC
www.fsc.org
MIX
Paper from
responsible sources
FSC™ C01624

For my mother Suzanne and my daughter Breyana,
for teaching me what is most important in life.
~ Ena Sabih

This book is dedicated to my wonderful wife Jennifer and my two
beautiful girls Lydia and Isabel. They make my life more complete
and more interesting. I am a blessed man to have the love
of them and the love of God.
~ Alfredo Escobar

Thank you to everyone who contributed to this book, especially Dr. Bénédicte Fontaine-Bisson for her review of the nutritional content. Thank you to my loving husband, my family and my friends for their support and encouragement throughout this project. A special thank you to a remarkable team who collaborated so generously to create this book. I am forever grateful for their guidance, time, and talents.

~ Ena Sabih

Did you eat your **vitamins** today?

You need them for energy, to grow, and to play.

Vitamins are found in foods we eat,

But they are all different and really neat.

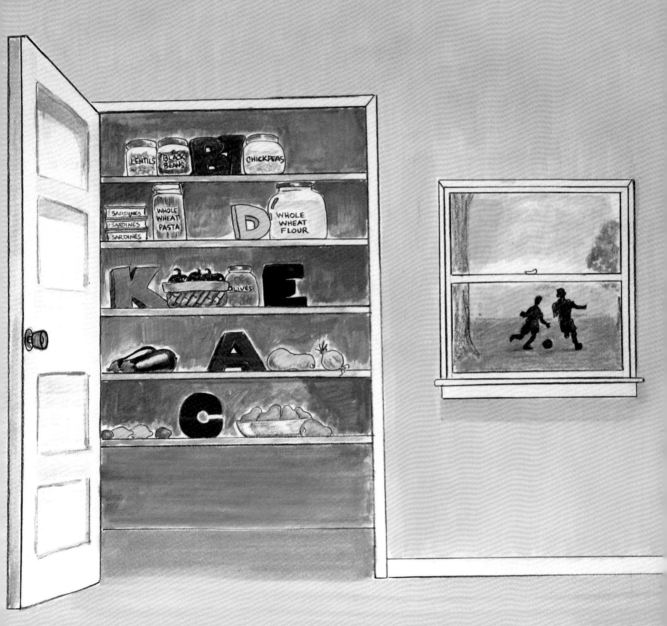

Sources of **vitamin A** for healthy eyes and skin,
Are orange fruits and vegetables like papaya and pumpkin.
Mangoes and squash also have what you need,
As do the carrots that grow from a seed.

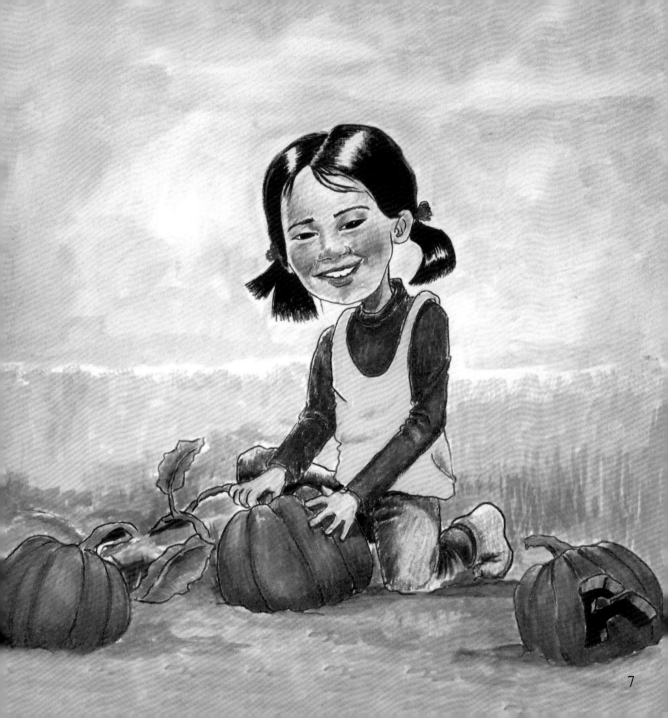

The **B vitamins** are quite complex;

Each one as important as the next.

They are good for your nerves and for your brain.

They're found in some vegetables, fish, and whole grains.

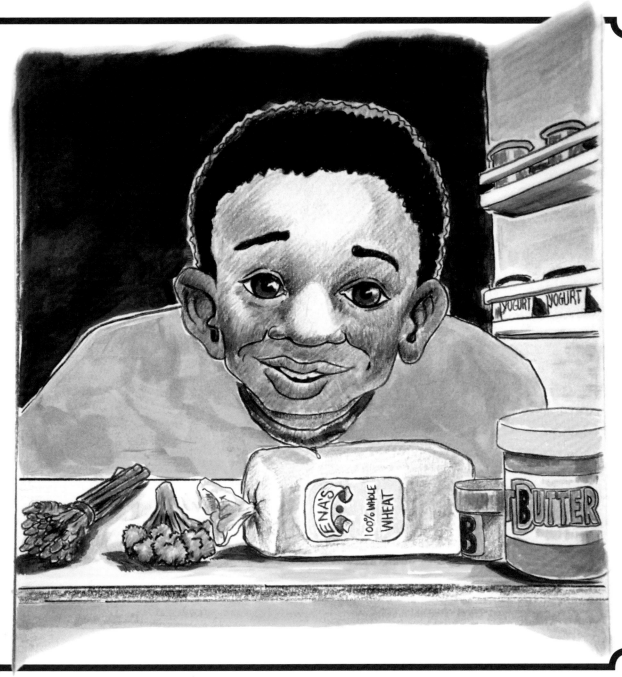

9

Vitamin C will help you fight the flu.
It's found in bell peppers and strawberries too.
It's in citrus fruit such as orange and lime
And helps heal your body, time after time.

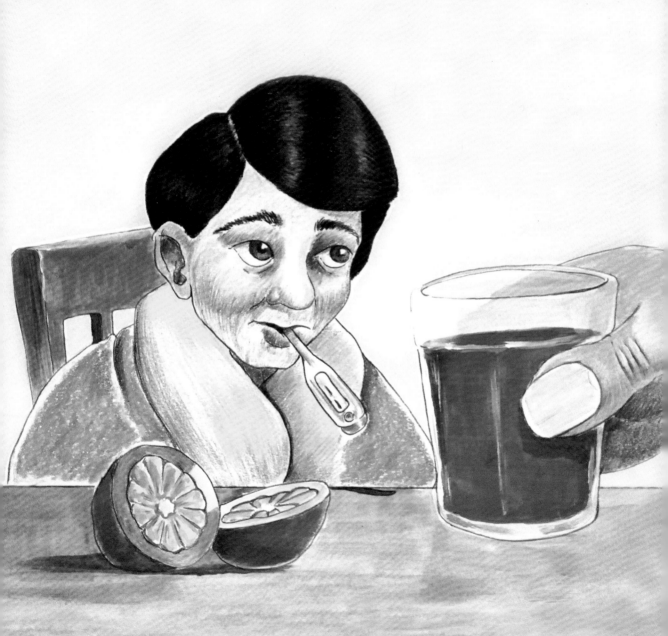

Sunshine on your skin makes **vitamin D,**

Which helps make your bones strong and healthy.

So play outside, move around, and have fun,

But remember the rules about being in the sun.

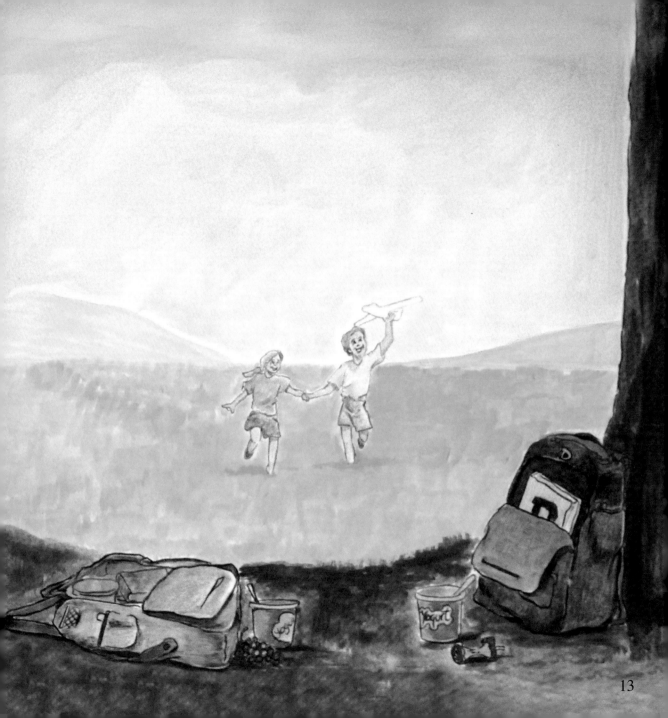

13

Vitamin E is in several seeds and oils
And in a few vegetables that grow in the soil.
It helps to protect your cells; that's what it can do.
So how about a serving of spinach for you?

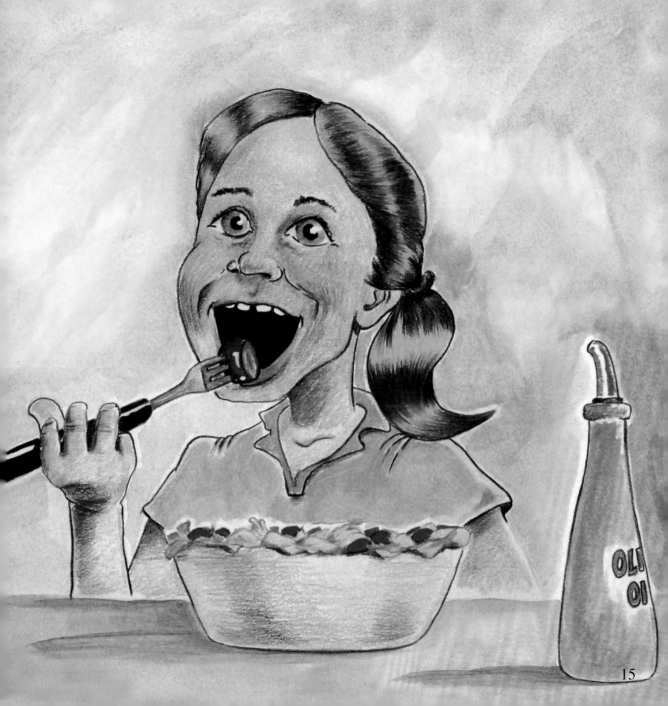

Vitamin K will help your cuts to stop bleeding,

So leafy green veggies are what you'll be needing.

It helps keep your bones healthy - to stand strong and tall

And helps prevent them from breaking, if ever you fall.

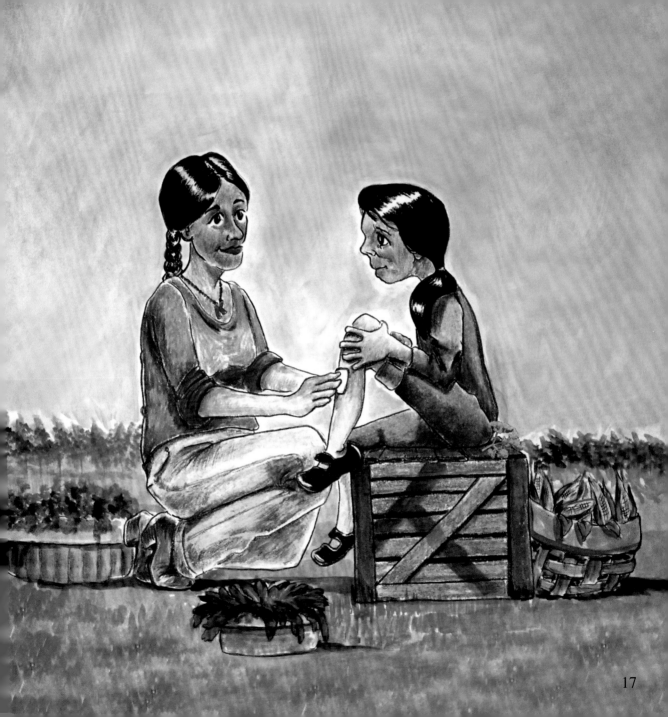

17

These next two vitamins are not known as letters.

Biotin and **folate** can make your body feel better.

They are, in fact, B vitamins too,

And here are some details on what they can do.

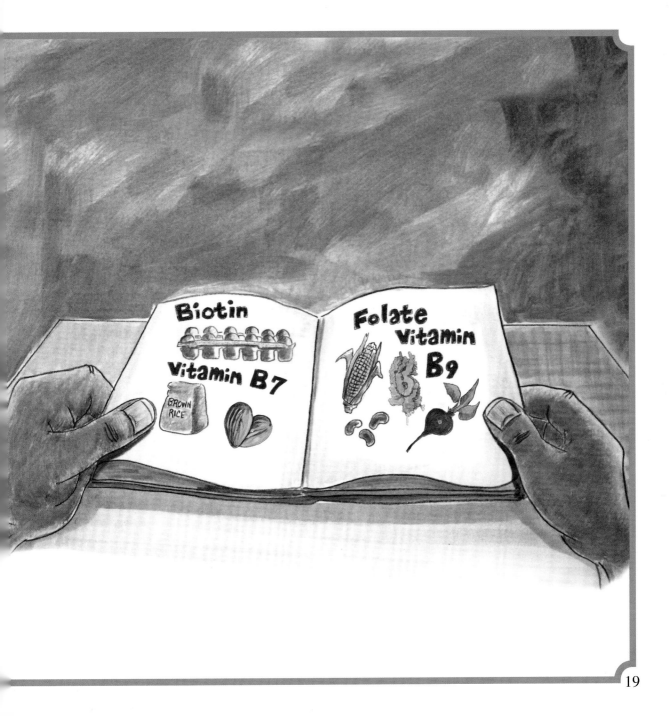

Biotin helps make energy, healthy skin and hair,
And here's something interesting, something rather rare.
It's made in the body; it's also found at the store.
If you buy brown rice or eggs, you'll have a little more.

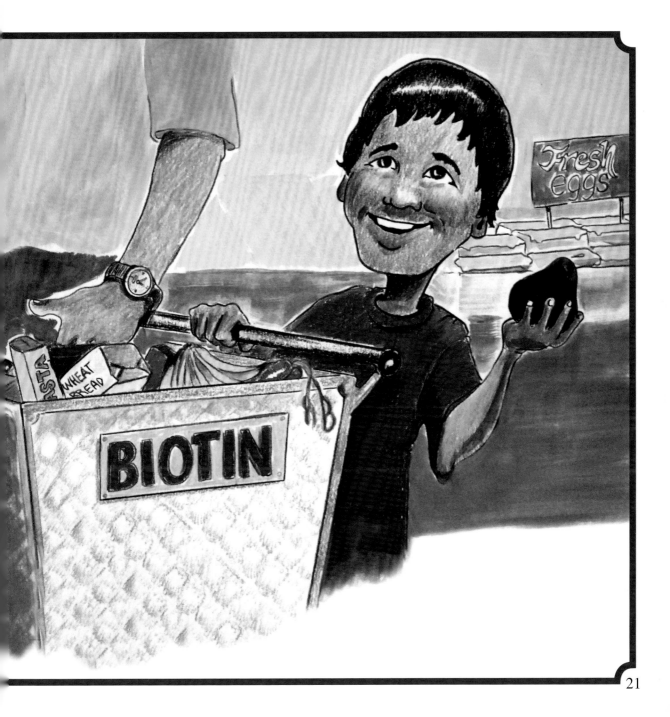

Folate is in many foods, like beans, kale, and corn.

It's important for development, before you're even born.

It comes from the word *foliage; leaves* is what it means.

So when you're hungry for a snack - don't forget the greens!

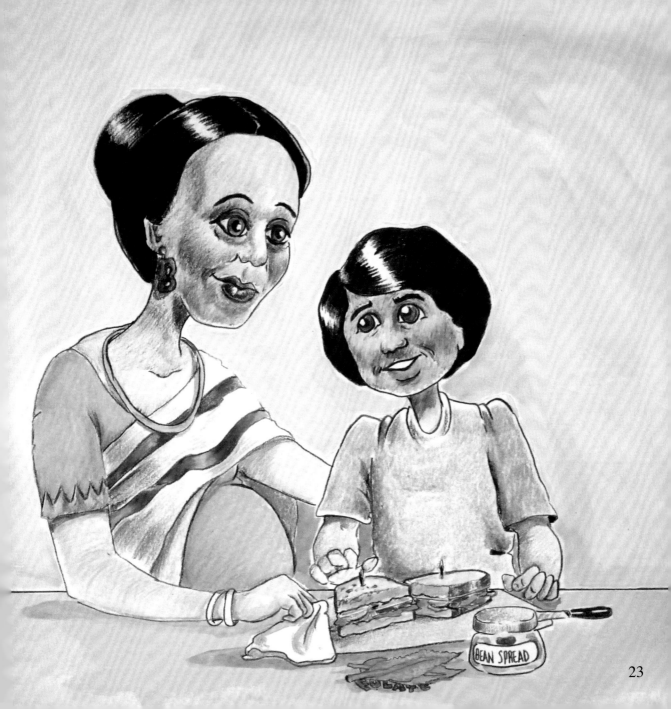

It's important to get your **vitamins** each day.

They help keep all kinds of diseases away.

They may also help you to think smart thoughts,

To learn, invent, and imagine a lot.

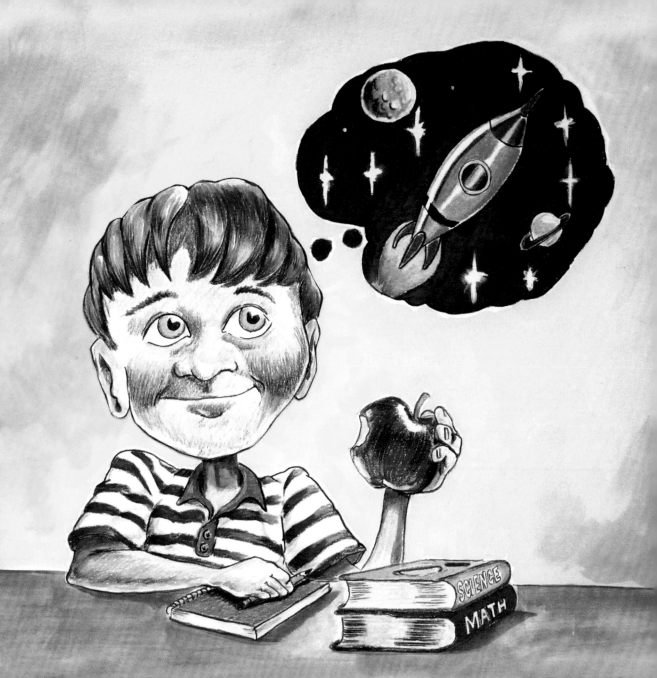

Enjoy natural foods; there are many to eat.

You'll find they are nature's special treat.

They're good for you and help keep you strong,

Just as parents have said all along.

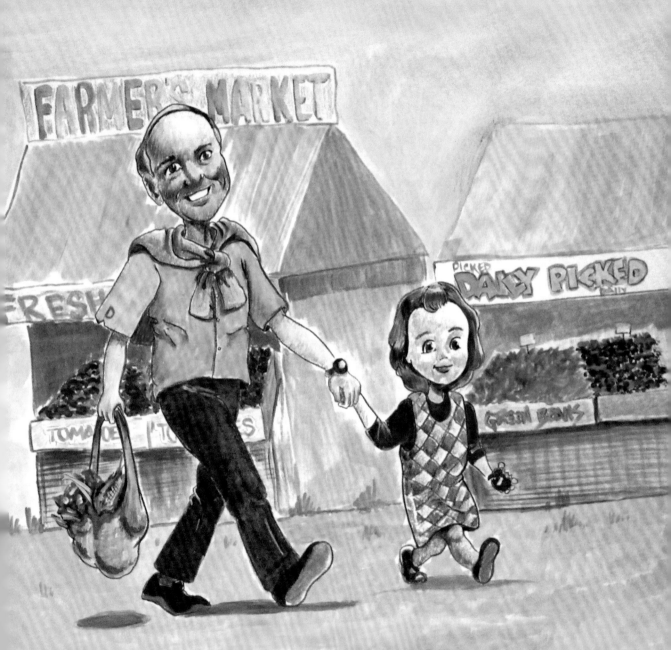

So be brave and try something new,

Even if it seems weird or yucky to you.

Perhaps you might like it. It could taste quite yummy.

Your parents will be grateful and so will your tummy.

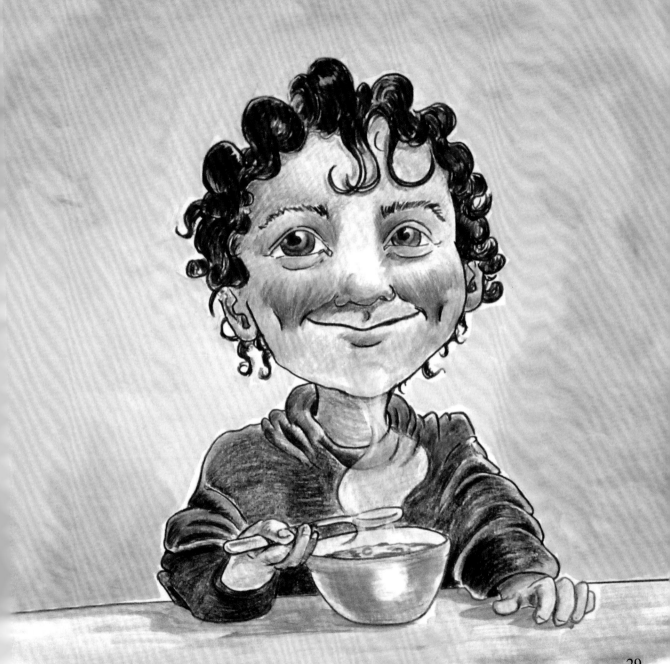

How about some barley, fennel, or berries?

Or maybe chickpeas, kale, or fresh cherries?

Perhaps some lentils or sweet potato?

Quinoa, kiwi, or the famous tomato?

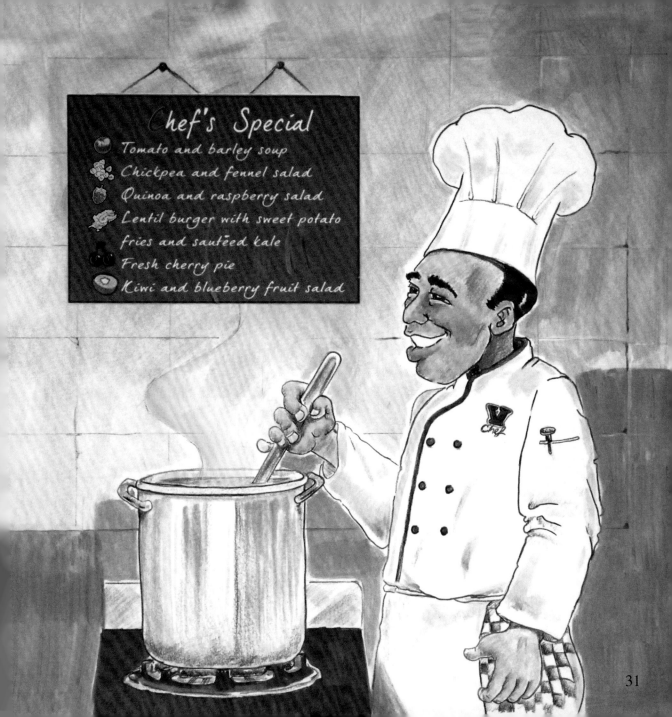

Have them at a picnic and every family meal,

Also from your lunchbox - this would be ideal.

No matter where you live, the city or the town,

Be sure to eat healthy foods and get your **vitamins** down.

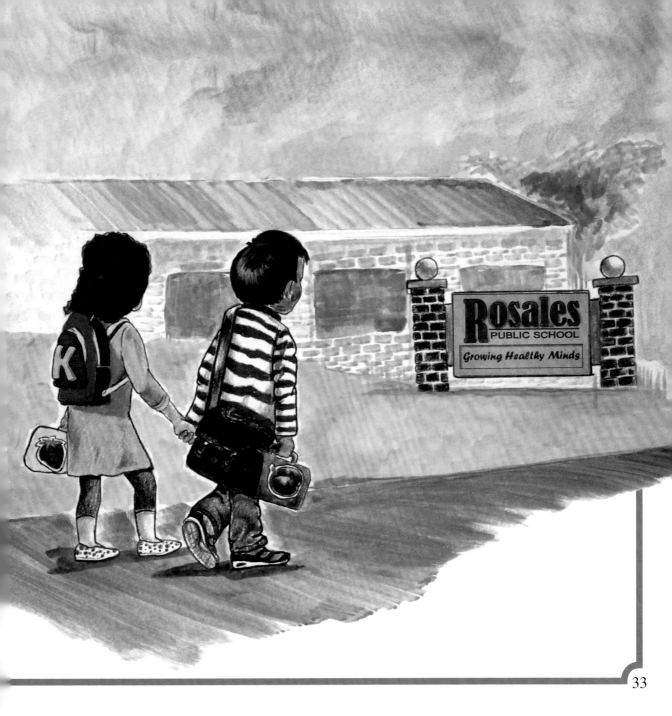

Think long and hard about the foods you eat,
And how **vitamins** work from your head to your feet.
Nutritious whole foods can help in many ways
To feel great and grow strong, day after day.

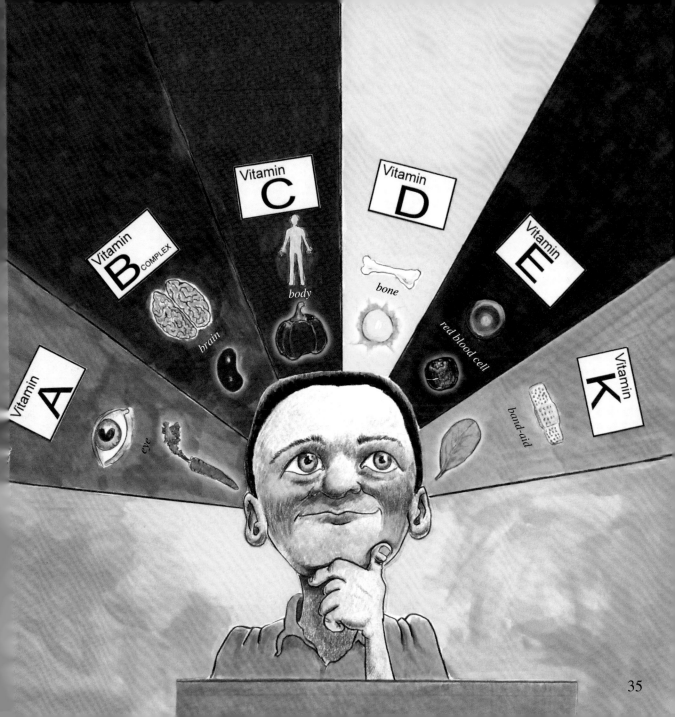

... Search and Find Activities ...

Search throughout the illustrations of this book to identify the following foods, as well as the vitamin letter A, B, C, D, E, and K. There is at least one letter in each illustration.

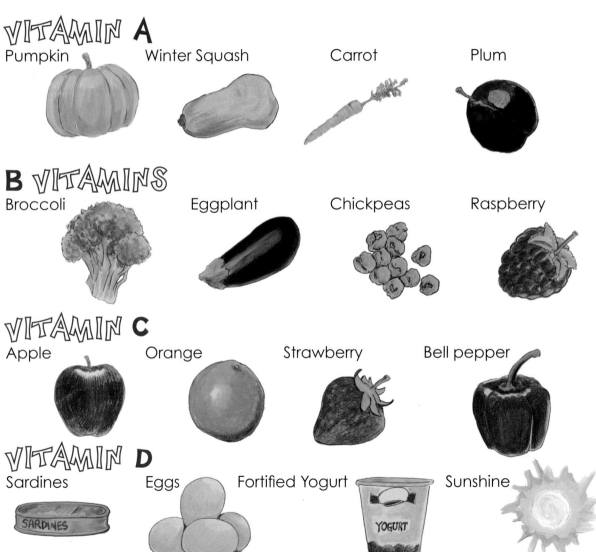

VITAMIN A

Pumpkin   Winter Squash   Carrot   Plum

B VITAMINS

Broccoli   Eggplant   Chickpeas   Raspberry

VITAMIN C

Apple   Orange   Strawberry   Bell pepper

VITAMIN D

Sardines   Eggs   Fortified Yogurt   Sunshine

SARDINES

YOGURT

VITAMIN E

Tomato Spinach Olive Oil Blueberries

VITAMIN K

Kale Parsley Asparagus Green Beans

BIOTIN (B7)

Onion Whole Wheat Bread Almonds Avocado

FOLATE (B9)

Romaine Lettuce Beet Beans Corn

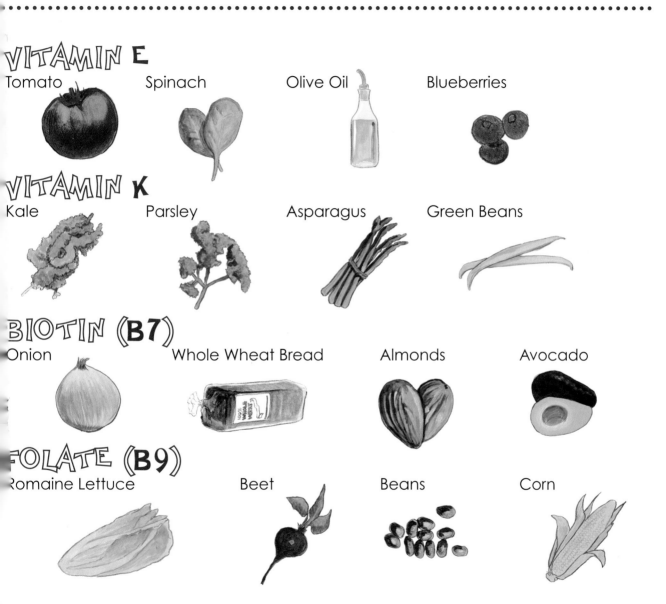

The answers to the search and find can be found on page 40.

Vitamins, Food Sources, and Discussion Questions

The following section provides additional information on vitamins and their food sources. It also offers some question for discussion. You may wish to refer back to the corresponding page and illustration for each vitamin, when reading the additional text and discussing the questions provided. Notice how one food can be a source of many vitamins

 ## VITAMIN A

Orange fruits and vegetables have beta-carotene, which your body can use to make vitamin A. Beta carotene is also found in other brightly coloured fruits and vegetables such as kale and tomatoes. The vitamin A found in foods that come from animal sources, such as eggs, fish, and yogurt, is ready for you body to use.

What is vitamin A good for?
What are your favorite orange fruits and vegetables?
If you had a garden what foods would you grow?

 ## B VITAMINS

There are several B vitamins including B1, B2, B3, B5, B6, B12, biotin and folate. Together they are referred to as the vitamin B-complex. Some of the B vitamins help to make energy from the food you eat. Other help to keep your skin, hair, and nerves healthy. Asparagus, cabbage, whole grains, and lentils all have some B vitamins.

What are some of the ways B vitamins help to keep your body healthy?
What fruits and vegetables do you like to eat?
Is there a fruit or vegetable in this book that you have never tried?

 ## VITAMIN C

Have you ever had an infection or caught the flu? Vitamin C helps your body fight bad bacteria an viruses. It is also important for healing. If you get hurt, vitamin C will help your body heal itself. Kiwifru papaya, and broccoli are other sources of vitamin C.

Why is vitamin C good for you?
How many citrus fruits can you name?
Why do you think there are so many fruits and vegetables with so many different colours and tastes?

.... 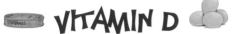 **VITAMIN D**   ....

Vitamin D is sometimes called the "sunshine vitamin". When the rays of the sun shine on your skin, your body makes vitamin D. Too much time in the sun can be harmful for your skin and can cause sunburns. Vitamin D is found in some foods such as eggs and sardines.

Why is vitamin D important for your body?
What are some of your favorite outdoor activities?
What are some sun safety rules?

.... 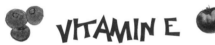 **VITAMIN E**   ....

Vitamin E protects our cells from damage. It is found in many oils, seeds, and nuts. Some of the vegetables that have vitamin E are olives, avocados, and tomatoes. Fruits, such as papayas, kiwifruits, and blueberries also have some vitamin E.

How does vitamin E help your body?
Do you like to eat salads?
What ingredients can you put in a salad?

.... 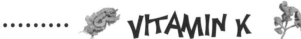 **VITAMIN K**  ....

Vitamin K is sometimes called the "band-aid" vitamin. If you get a cut, it will help stop the bleeding. It also plays an important role in maintaining healthy bones. It is found in green leafy vegetables such as spinach and romaine lettuce.

Why is vitamin K important for you?
Have you ever been to a farm to pick fruits or vegetables?
What foods are grown locally, where you live?

BIOTIN (Vitamin B7)

Biotin is made in your body by the bacteria that live in your intestines. It is needed to keep your skin and hair healthy. Biotin is found in some nuts, yogurt, and cauliflower.

Why is biotin important for your body?
Do you ever go shopping for food?
What types of food does your family like to eat?

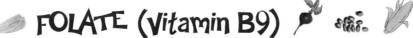# FOLATE (Vitamin B9)

Folate was important for the development of your brain and spinal cord when you were growing in your mother's tummy. It is found in leafy "greens" such as spinach and cabbage. It is also found in many types of beans.

Why do you need folate?
Do you like to cook?
What are some things you can do to help out with meals at home?